MW00824926

What are We Going to Do about Mom and Dad?

A Navigational Guide to Senior Living and Care

JANE MEYERS-BOWEN

ISBN 978-1-54398-474-3 eBook 978-1-54398-475-0

This book is dedicated to all my friends, colleagues, managers and family members who have taken a stand for me. Your support and inspiration have made a difference.

Special thanks to my husband for your endless love and always believing in me;

To my friends Claudia Glaze and Cynthia Graham for hours of editing and years of sisterhood;

To all the seniors and their families for teaching me about the richness of the last chapters in life.

CONTENTS

Goals of This Book

1. Educate adult children about recognizing and addressing the aging issues of their parents.

2. Provide supportive coaching for adult children as they take on significant new roles and responsibilities during a time of major transition for the senior in their lives.

3. Determine the different risks, solutions, and finally the rewards of a happy and safe parent.

Most of us don't know much about senior living and care until we are confronted with a parent whose mental, physical, cognitive, or emotional health changes. However, a recent Pew Research survey finds that 14% of adults in their 40s and 50s have already cared for an aging parent or other elderly family member, and nearly seven-in-ten say that it is "very" (48%) or "somewhat" (20%) likely they will have to do this in the future.

I have written this book as a guide for families of seniors, seniors themselves, neighbors, friends and ministers – anyone in a position to assist a senior in a major life transition. As a former nurse who has worked in retirement and assisted living communities for over fifteen years, I have had the opportunity and responsibility of coaching over four thousand seniors and their families with making wise decisions regarding senior living and care. I was honored to be present and involved in such an important process.

Experience is the best teacher. I have also had to deal with this issue in my own life with my parents and in-laws. Let me tell you about my story that happened before I was professionally involved with seniors and their families. Before I was professionally involved with senior living, our family faced a major wake up call. It was July, and we were heading for a family reunion in Montana. Excited about seeing my parents face to face, we arrived late and got up early to join them for breakfast. The conversation flowed. We got updated and shared a few laughs and discussed the plan for the day.

My mother and father had driven over the Rocky Mountains, with Dad at the wheel; they had arrived the day before. He owned a small trucking company before World War II, drove troop trucks during the war throughout Europe, and later bought and operated a 10,000-acre farm, which required his driving heavy equipment and trucks. So, Dad was the trusted driver in our family.

Several years before, Dad had open heart bypass surgery. He was always very bright, not much of a talker, a man of confidence. However, he emerged from surgery a different person. When he came out of recovery, my sister-in-law (who was also a nurse) and I looked at each other and were startled by his notable cognitive changes. He wasn't as alert and was somewhat disoriented and confused. We quickly assumed or wanted to believe it was something temporary. We later learned that it is not uncommon for an underlying Alzheimer's condition to become obvious after heart surgery.

We watched him struggle to come back to normalcy after the surgery with exercise and diet changes, and we did see some improvement. Unfortunately, this progress cemented our denial, and life went on as usual. When I observed my father's mental state toward the end of that day in July months later, I realized that Dad was in serious mental decline. He was disengaged, not following the conversation, and seemed confused. I took my mother aside and said, "Mom, things are pretty serious with Dad. How did he drive the car across the Rocky Mountains?" The floodgates opened. In her own pain, fear, and tired spirit she confirmed what they had been trying to deny and hide…Dad had mid-stage dementia, later diagnosed as Alzheimer's Disease. Families tend to focus on the _identified patient_. In this case, my father. However, my mother was also suffering from lack of sleep, because Dad would get up in the middle of the night, get in the car, and drive half a block from home and get lost. She was losing weight with all her worry. Unfortunately, we all lived hundreds of miles away, and their friends had slowed down calling on them. Worst of all, Mom couldn't bring herself to admit it was all too much for her to handle by herself and felt guilty at the prospect of placing Dad in a care facility.

So started my family's journey to help both my mom and dad. Although my dad's change of condition was mental, it was as difficult for us as it is for other families dealing with mobility issues, depression, and nutritional challenges. My own family's experience later provided the inspiration for my professional move to senior living. Making this important lifestyle change as stress-free as possible for the senior and those that support them became such meaningful work for me. I found I was in the position to help create a fulfilling last chapter in people's lives. The advice that I share comes from my personal and professional experience. I have also referenced the valuable work of others as well. Please keep in mind that I urge you to get medical, legal and financial advice as you address each of your specific situations. This book comes from being on the ground

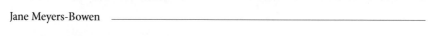

on a day by day basis. I hope this book helps you and your family's journey to be a positive one.

Chapter One

OMG What Happened?

The Truth About Aging

Many times, the changes in our elderly relatives (parent, grandparent, aunt, uncle, neighbor, or friend) are very subtle. They show up as an unexplained dent in the car, questionable "phone friends," mail stacking up, and not attending church services or family celebrations any longer.

Family members witnessing their parents' emerging fragility (even when it is ever so slight) challenges our own view of ourselves. The role reversal from child to caregiver forces a set of responsibilities that are complex and are fraught with feelings of loss, fear, guilt, and uncertainty.

Facing the aging problem of our parent(s) or older adult can be one of the most powerful experiences of life. It presses us up against ourselves as well as the family system. Old sibling rivalries, money and power issues, and other unresolved anger, guilt, and loss reemerge. And I'm not sure we are ever really ready! Having assisted thousands of families and seniors to navigate this life experience, I can share some strategies than can take some of the wear and tear out of the process and hopefully offer you some sound how-tos that will hopefully provide some joy, compassion, personal growth and help you forge a new relationship with someone you love.

Aging is one of those subjects that terrifies Americans. Seniors in their sixties and above have enjoyed a place of power and authority in our culture and the world. They have rewritten the rules in fashion, politics, music, health, and business. Today, Baby Boomers yearn to be forever young. However, the fear of growing old handicaps us all in dealing with our personal and our parents' aging problem.

Myths, False Assumptions, and Fake News about Aging

- "My mother can make her own decisions!" Yes, but recognize that making a major decision like moving out of their family home of sixty years may be more than she can handle. Ask her if she's ready to move, and her response will be "No, I'm not ready." Families want to honor their parents' dignity, which is very respectful.

    Often the real hidden concern about moving is "How am I going to get rid of my stuff?" whether it's in their house, attic, garage, or shop. Younger generations are probably not standing in line for the china. So, "all the stuff" is making the decision! The best advice is counter-intuitive. As young adults, we tend to take 80–90 percent of our stuff with us when we move. By necessity, when moving to a retirement home, most seniors are reducing the stuff they will take with them 75 – 80% percent. So, focusing on what they are going to take with them rather than worrying about what they are going to get rid of will simplify this move tremendously. Assure them you will handle "all the extra stuff" later. Some families have a "giving party" where members of the family choose even a small item like a tea cup. The most important part is to tell the story behind the tea cup.

- I can get by with a little help from my friends.

  Many families can end up focusing on the frail parent's needs without regard for the other parent, his/her spouse who has assumed twenty-four-hour caregiving responsibility for too long. Agingcare.com references that 30 percent of caregivers pass away before those they are caring for. Thus, the plan needs to take into account the whole system – both patient and caregiver spouse.

  Families that live across the country often rely on neighbors and friends to make sure their parents get to the grocery store, get to their doctor's appointments, and care for their pets. Sure, on a temporary basis this can be very workable, but at some point, this strategy is unfair, inappropriate at best, and not sustainable.

- Home is where the heart is!

  Is that a statement about bricks and mortar or where the memories are? Ensure that seniors are involved in choosing the things that represent their life. It could be family pictures, art work, souvenirs from their travel, or gifts they received from their spouse, children, parents, etc. that remind them of happy times in life.

- Mom is doing great!

  When seniors have maintained a healthy body and mind, family members can easily overlook their parents' loneliness, lack of sense of belonging, and their need to know that they are or can contribute to the world. Many seniors are involved with their communities and friends, but over time their friends move away or pass away, and neighborhoods change. Isolation takes its toll. Even with the most attentive family members, taking their parent to church and out to breakfast weekly takes about four hours. Let's assume, with twelve hours of awake time per day, that represents eighty-four hours of awake time. And if a parent doesn't talk to another person all week, that is eighty hours of alone time per week!

The other scenario is families are so busy running them to the grocery store, doctor's appointments, cleaning their home, preparing meals, fixing their fence, and writing their bills, they have little time to sit on the couch with their arm around them and listening to their favorite stories about their childhood, the war, and life when Hoover was President.

Traumatic events can tip the scale also. For example, loss of spouse or their driver's license, or loss of hearing and eyesight can leave them stranded at home. These traumatic events can start to erode one's overall health. Their world can shrink to just two to three rooms and sitting in front of the television. Slowly they lose muscle mass, which contributes to balance and strength issues, followed by social connection and confidence, and they start eating TV dinners. It can lead to a downward spiral where everything is fine until it's not.

- Mom and Dad are fine in their home.

  I think one of the biggest myths is to believe keeping your parents in their home is the absolute best situation. This could be a quality strategy for any given person, but there are many variables that affect the wisdom of this situation.

- I know what the future holds.

> Never promise your parents that you won't move them out of their home or to a nursing home! Many adult children's hands are tied when facing the realities. The burden of guilt is what takes the family down. *The only promise you should make is that you will do your best to see that they have the highest quality of life possible with the resources (human and otherwise) that you have available.*

Seniors are living longer. Thanks to the success of medical research on heart disease and cancer, seniors are healthier today. Forty years ago, seniors didn't have many options when they needed more care. If they weren't safe at home, they moved in with their children and later went to a nursing home for additional care. Today, there are several options! (See Chapter 3). However, even today seniors and families don't realize what is available. *Frankly, most of us don't go shopping for senior living and care until we need to, have to, or are forced to.*

Not only are there more options, but they are better, cleaner, and safer than twenty-five years ago. And today these options are more focused on health and wellbeing, not just custodial care.

Beginning the Journey . . . What's Ahead?

There are four key things you have to know as you assist a senior through this major life change.

1. Knowing this change will take some time (if you are not in a crisis),

2. Knowing what the options are,

3. Knowing that most seniors are empowered and legally protected to make their own decisions, and

4. Knowing that life isn't over for your loved one.

Facing urgent and unavoidable need for change can be very uncomfortable. These situations are few in life but can prove to be a time of great growth, excitement, and opportunity as well. Families reunite with each other and their parents in meaningful ways.

Chapter Two

Buckle Up...It could be a Bumpy Ride!

Most of us don't know much about senior living and care from my experience until we are confronted with a parent whose mental, physical, cognitive, social, or emotional health changes.

When families would come to investigate our retirement/assisted living community, my first question I ask myself is, *"What happened?"* Something propelled them into my office. Families are not always forthright about what-occurred. Be it a gradual or a rapid change, the denial has melted away. A new reality about their parent has emerged. It could be noticeable memory loss, complaints of loneliness, medication errors, symptoms of depression, an illness or injury that resulted in a hospitalization or changes in mobility, decision-making, social appropriateness, and/or emotional control. A doctor made the observation that their parent wasn't safe living alone anymore.

You may learn about these changes from visiting your parent during the holidays. Phone relationships are common today with families living far apart. Weekly phone calls don't always alert you to what is happening, and you are caught off guard. Or it could be a call from their neighbor voicing concern about your mother or father's wellbeing. Or you notice large sums of money disappearing from their bank account without explanation. You may even see unexplained bruises and bumps. Families often witness deterioration of property, of order in daily living, and questionable decision-making.

Families often encounter difficult times when taking their mother or father on a trip with them. A trip that is intended to bring stimulation, joy, and much-needed family time turns out to be one of the most stressful, yet revealing, experiences. Taking your parents out of their day-to-day world, which they know inside and out, puts them into a spin of confusion, disorientation, and anxiety. The fragility of their life structure that holds everything together for them becomes obvious.

All of a sudden, you are thrust into a new reality and are overwhelmed with the new responsibilities you now have and decisions that need to be made to keep your parent/senior safe.

Initially, a lot of cognitive and physical decline is written off as "Mom's getting older" and is disregarded as normal, within the norms, or nothing to worry about. A parent can present well or may be skilled in dodging, bobbing, and weaving the issues, laughing at the right times, looking to others to answer key questions, or giving false answers or reassurances. Denial may handicap your ability to see the truth. Wanting to respect your parents' dignity, you assume your parents need to and can make decisions about their own lives. Stop! It is time to examine the evidence you see. Delay and denial can mean the difference between a timely, smooth transition and a crisis-driven decision, making it rough on everyone.

When is the time for a change?

For each person it can be a different time. Loneliness can be the biggest motivator to move to a more vibrant living situation. The loss of a spouse or family moving away can dramatically impact the quality of one's life. Unfortunately, many times it's when there's a 911 call, figuratively or literally. It could be a fall, an injury, a financial disaster, or a medical situation as common as severe dehydration or a common UTI (urinary tract infection). Whatever the cause, the solution will involve change. My advice is to get on the road and start the journey. Do your best to see this trip as an adventure for your loved one that could lead to greater health and well-being for them and peace of mind for you.

Let Freedom Ring

The one of the greatest fears seniors face is losing their freedom, which predisposes them to not ask for help.

Nobody wants to lose their independence. So, working through this process of change is usually not going to be a walk in the park. Today's seniors don't roll over easily. Yet, most don't realize that institutional life is limited to only the highest levels of care. Many senior living communities offer so much control of their personal decisions. For example, they can decide when they eat, what they eat, when they go to bed and get up, and even when they come and go. Yes, there are some restrictions on what you wear in the common areas (no pajamas in the dining room) and basic etiquette is required. Ironically, seniors enjoy more freedom in their lives when freed up from cooking, cleaning, yard work, and home maintenance, as they have more time to be with family and friends, focus on their health (not just their illnesses), and do their personal work, like figuring out their legacy.

Understandably, we all typically dig our heels in unless we understand the need for change. The need for change can be driven by the fact that their environment is no longer safe and no longer supports their wellbeing.

What Are the Dangers?

If a senior's home is filled with stairs, scatter rugs, and extension cords, with no walk-in shower available, he/she is at a greater risk of a debilitating injury every single day.

A senior can become a target for crime. If the neighborhood has gone downhill or one's home and yard show signs of disrepair, your parent may become more vulnerable to being taken advantage of.

A senior with mobility and balance issues, diminishing vision, or changes in memory and cognitive abilities may no longer be safe in even the best environment. Whether it is taking medications accurately, giving up step stools/ladders, managing finances, or scheduling (and remembering) doctor's appointments, keeping up becomes extremely stressful. At some point it becomes necessary for you to step into their life in a new, caring way. Most seniors don't want to be a bother or burden and won't ask for help even when they really need it. Even though they might not admit it, an intervention from you may secretly be a welcome relief.

An agile and clear-minded senior who is living in the best neighborhood but is no longer able to drive can suffer from many hours of being alone and feeling cut off from others.

Generally speaking, the best living situation is not the most restrictive one but the most independent setting that is safe. Most seniors find that a well-chosen senior community, where their basic living and social needs are provided, offers them more independence, not less.

As families gear up to facilitate this life transition, there is much to do.

A Roadmap for This Journey

Step 1: Assemble a team.

Handling this process single-handedly is very challenging if not impossible, especially if you are living very full lives at home and work and are facing your own health issues and financial challenges.

There are many people that can help, including your parents' neighbors, trusted physician, minister, professional care manager, referral agency, government agencies, and senior friends. The A-team is likely to consist of immediate family members.

For example, here is a list of tasks to be shared or delegated.

Team responsibilities	Person	Date to be completed
Organizer/Communicator		
Financial researcher (Meet with Financial Planner, Realtor etc.)		
Senior Living and Care Options researcher		
Packer		
Mover		
Unpacker		
Logistics lead (forwarding mail, finding new doctor, setting up new phone, etc.)		
Disposal of unneeded clothing, furniture, home décor, etc.		
Interface with Mom and Dad		
Celebration planner		
Other		

Remember . . .

In baseball each player has a position, but as soon as the ball is hit by the batter, everyone on the field starts moving playing their primary role or in a backup position to support other players. Placing people in the right position, utilizing their strengths, agreeing on a set of ground rules that everyone plays by, and keeping eyes on the ball, i.e., the senior's wellbeing, will generally result in a smoother transition.

Senior Rights

Often family members want to take over things or feel obligated to figure out what is right for their senior.

Today, seniors have rights about their lives under federal and state laws. In the state of Washington, the legislature identifies the <u>rights of choice</u> (make one's own decisions about life and care), <u>participation</u> (being actively involved in the decision-making process), <u>privacy</u>, and the <u>opportunity to engage</u> in religious, political, civic, recreational, and other social activities. Vulnerable adults living in long-term-care facilities or seniors in the community at large have access to adult protective services and ombudsmen, advocates who can assist them in protecting their rights. By and large, seniors are deemed competent to conduct their own affairs. The family may have to work within that context, i.e., assisting them by exercising patience, love, and compassion. Even with a designated power of attorney, the senior remains the decision-maker unless they are unable to do so, e.g., if they are incapacitated. It may be determined by the courts that a specific individual requires a legal guardian to act on their behalf. Powers of attorney are only actionable while the individual is alive.

Step Two: Gather the information you need.

- Know your senior

  A conversation with your loved one's physician about the type and appropriate level of care is crucial as you begin to look at the options. Having this information will allow for a quick paring-down of the list to include only the organizations that can meet the needs of your senior.

Pause for a moment. Describe your parent's modus operandi. Is he/she organized, happy, groomed or messy, clumsy, or a bit disheveled? Is he/she quiet, hesitant, apprehensive, angry, absent-minded, friendly, socially confident, articulate? It's important to first understand their baseline. Being any of those doesn't indicate much. But if their current behavior rapidly changes

Physical		Emotional		Cognitive		Social	
Weight loss	✓	Fear of being alone		Not taking meds per doctor's orders		Friendship with unusual people	
Multiple falls	✓	Wearing pajamas all day		Unpaid bills or Mountains of unopened mail		Stopped calling friends	
Unexplained injuries		Feeling despondent	✓	Loss of money or Questionable financial decisions	✓	Stopped participating in things previously enjoyed	
Unkempt appearance		Becoming secretive		Pets not cared for		Trusting strangers with entry into home	
Home & yard in disarray	✓	Becoming paranoid	✓	Vehicle accumulating dents		Disclosing personal information to strangers	✓
Sleeping too much or too little	✓	Frequently calling in distress; call 911		Food or meds beyond pull dates		Loss of social confidence	
Tremors or Walks with a shuffle.		Talks of wanting to die.	✓	Up on the roof cleaning the gutters.		Complaints of not feeling loved.	

from their norm, it may indicate a change of condition and suggest a trend downward. Many things can influence how we feel, think, or move about. It's important to seek out a doctor's opinion. Urinary tract infections are often first recognized by confusion. Over medication, old medication, or no medication can be the culprits. Vitamin deficiencies, depression, and unmanaged pain can affect sleep patterns, appetite, and peace of mind.

Warning signals- Check ✔ for each applicable parameter.

Look for warning signals that can be overlooked or rationalized away. This may be a good exercise to share with other family members.

Step Three: How are we going to pay for this?

The third step is to figure out where the senior stands financially. Many older adults keep a tight lip and grip on their finances. Getting an accurate view of their assets and liabilities will define a certain number of options available or unavailable to them.

Financial statement

Total assets	Asset value	Total liabilities	Liability
Large & fixed assets Equity in home, vehicles		Long term liabilities (mortgage, equity loans, reverse mortgages, and car loans)	
Liquid assets- Investment accounts Cash on hand (in bank and under the mattress)		Short term liabilities Credit card debt Hospital bills	
Personal items (cars, equipment, tools)			
Jewelry, gun collection, art collection, etc.			
Total			
Total net worth			

Let's take a closer look at each of these factors.

Home equity

Most seniors fund their retirement living and/or assisted care with the equity of their homes. However, look for draws against it or if they had taken out a reverse mortgage, which is senior program for borrowing money against the equity. Both scenarios could erode a substantial portion of their equity. Also, reverse mortgages can require the owners to occupy their residence.

Investments

Often when older adults get into their eighties or nineties, their investment portfolios may have been drained. Also, seniors that over-invested in equity funds could have taken a beating in the early 2000s or during the crash in 2008, without adequate time to re-build. On the other hand, many bought Microsoft for a song too!

Personal items

Collections may have grown in value or become worthless. Antique appraisers can help evaluate, price, and place antiques in the market. It is important to contact a reputable appraiser who has an expertise in the type of products you are trying to sell, be it firearms, jewelry, pottery, Asian art, etc. *https://www.isa-appraisers.org/find-an-appraiser

Other Possible Funding Options

Long-term care insurance

In the late 1970s, a fairly new insurance product was sold to seniors as Nursing Home Insurance often with lifetime coverage once meeting the requirements for care. As the industry of senior living and care started to explode with new care options (we will discuss those in Chapter Three), many insurance companies accepted using their policies to pay for assisted living services, which was a less expensive care option and more appropriately met seniors' needs as most didn't need high-level nursing care but only assistance with activities of daily living (ADLs). So it appeared as a win-win situation for seniors, insurance companies, and assisted living operators. However, in time, a number of insurance companies dropped their long-term insurance line of business dramatically, complaining that actuaries underestimated how long people would live.

If your senior has purchased a long-term care policy, it's time to evaluate this option. With your senior present, call the insurance company and ask for the underwriting department to "start a claim" versus calling the customer service department. You will be assured of more accurate information regarding their specific policy.

- Questions to ask the underwriting department:

    1. What is the daily benefit (total dollar value of funds)?

    2. How many months will it pay out (older policies paid out for life, but most pay out over two to five years)?

    3. Once a claim has been accepted, is there a waiting period (often you will see a sixty to ninety day waiting period)?

    4. Do you have to continue to pay premiums (most policies don't require this)?

    5. How many ADLs are required and which ones are recognized (usually two to three)? Activities of daily living (ADLs) are defined as assistance with medication management, bathing, dressing, grooming, toileting, and escorting. A nursing assessment by the insurance company will be required to determine the needs. Most seniors need help with medications and bathing in the beginning. (Some insurance

companies don't count medication management as an ADL— they can be rascals!)

Life insurance policies

Unfortunately, many seniors have cancelled their life insurance policy long ago. For example, it may have been a twenty-year-term life contract that had to be fulfilled, or the premiums became prohibitive with whole life policies and seniors will have dropped the insurance. Life insurance's purpose has been to protect families during the early years.

However, some life insurance policies have a cash value that can be used for assisted living care *prior to death under certain conditions.*

Also, there is a growing secondary market for selling life insurance policy contracts for a much greater amount than the cash surrender value the insurance company will pay. Someone will buy the contract and make the payments, and when the person dies the death benefit will be paid out to the new party. Thus, both strategies can free up some cash for care needs today.

Government programs

Many families are confused with the difference between Medicare and Medicaid.

Medicaid pays for assistance with ADLs. Medicaid is a joint relationship between state and federal government. Not all state Medicare programs pay for care. Medicare pays for ongoing medical expenses (doctor, hospital, etc.) and is used to pay for short-term care in a skilled nursing facility or rehabilitation facility for a qualifying illness, an injury, or home healthcare (visiting nurse services, physical, speech, and/or occupational therapy.). It does not pay for custodial long-term care, including rent for a retirement/assisted living community. Currently, however, there is discussion about Medicare pay or some home support in the future.

Unfortunately, with the slashing of government reimbursement rates, fewer and fewer assisted living communities have Medicaid contracts. Those that do have a Medicaid contract operate in several different ways. Some will have a direct admission program and while others may have a spend-down program.

The direct admission program requires verification that your older adult needs help with a number of specified ADLs and has been accepted to receive Medicaid. Typically, there is a ceiling for income, and they can have only $2000 in assets. Most have a five-year look-back period to ensure that seniors are not hiding their assets.

Typically, the higher quality communities have a spend-down program of one to three years that requires the senior to use their private funds as long as they have them. Then when the seniors spend down to meet Medicaid requirements, they are accepted on a state paid program. Often the state requires apartment sharing. Social Security benefits go toward their rent and care, but residents get a small amount of money for personal incidentals.

The government offers some affordable housing programs too that promote the building of moderate-income independent apartments. These programs are called bond programs and tax credit programs. The government guarantees loans for builders as construction funds at a favorable rate with the stipulation that at least 20 percent of the apartments are reserved for people with lower incomes. The benefit for seniors is a lower-than-market-rate for an apartment, and they can still have some assets, allowing them to stretch their dollars.

Aid and Attendance for Wartime Veterans

This benefit was initially funded in the early 1950s. Few people really knew much about it until the investigative news show, *60 Minutes*, broadcast a program in 2004. Structured very differently from Medicaid but often confused with it, many people assumed they did not qualify. Unlike Medicaid, the veteran or spouse can still have some assets (within reason). This program was put in place to help stretch the assets of a veteran to address any care needs they may have developed in their senior years. This program also provides benefits for a surviving spouse upon the death of the veteran. https://www.veteranaid.org/apply.php

If your parent actively served during official wartime (not necessarily in battle or overseas), had an honorable discharge, and is over sixty-five years old, they may qualify for this benefit. They have to verify with their physician that they need assistance with a certain number of ADLs. There will be a three-year look back to ensure that their funds weren't given to family members as a way to hide their assets. There are two steps in the application process. The first is a short form and starts the clock. The second is the full application, which requires a lot of documentation, including their military discharge papers, birth, death, marriage certificates, bank statements, etc. If the veteran qualifies for benefits, they pay retroactively to the date of the short form application.

Family Contribution

Many seniors really don't think they would live as long as they do. They save money their whole lives, live conservatively, and are living five to ten years longer than they figured they would. Families are often called upon to help out. A case in point is my mother-in-law Susie who lived to age ninety-five. She wasn't on any meds, suffered no dementia, and lived alone in a three-story condo until she was eighty-eight. When she wanted to move closer to family, we found her a community that had the moderate-income program (a unique HUD program that provides low cost construction loans to the operator in return for some apartments reserved for people with moderate income), which helped conserve the funds she had. Her son and daughter paid her a monthly stipend, and they put it out to our greater family that we all had to help Grandma. It was a rich family experience, and even our younger children, who were nine and ten at the time, gave her a couple of dollars from their allowance to do their part. Not everyone contributed.

Not everyone could. Not everyone wanted to. But I guess that's life in the big city.

When someone's family is not available or able, I have worked with a few seniors whose church has provided some financial help and in one case a fraternal organization provided a stipend to help with the costs of care.

It's always a good idea to consult a financial advisor to assess how long one's money will last. For planning purposes, you will want to note that most facilities will have yearly rental rate increase from 2–7 percent. Most will not commit to it in the lease, but you can ask what the annual history of rate increases has been. Often the market will determine the rental rate increases.

Chapter Three

Moving Ahead

Now that you have done an initial assessment, consulted with the physician, banker, financial planner, etc., and assembled a team of support, it's time to move into action.

*What Are the Senior Living & Care Options? Taking a Closer Look**

Living options	Positives	Negatives
Stay at home with help Help may come from family or professionals. On-going care provided by families can greatly impact the family's employment, financial resources and personal health. Home care is when outside caregivers come daily or several times a week. They provide non-medical care: bathing, dressing, grooming, cooking, cleaning, transportation, etc.. Professional home care companies are regulated by state laws and do background checks on caregivers. Professional home care companies usually require a minimum number of hours per care trip. An hourly rate of $20–$35 × 2–3 hours × number of days per week– these fees can add up fast. Home Health care provide help with medications, wound care, physical, occupational and speech therapy.	*Most seniors want to stay in their homes and probably will. Assuming seniors remain healthy and their homes are not riddled with stairs, it continues to be a very good choice. Changes of condition, hanging up the car keys, and changes in the neighborhood can trigger a time to re-evaluate. *Being close to their support communities, i.e., neighbors, doctors, churches, friends, etc., seniors stay active, involved, and contributing. *Depending on the financial resources, bringing in help with home & yard needs, personal care, transportation, etc. can help to stay "independent" at home. Help can be a family member that moves in, a renter to share the costs/tasks, a professional personal care provider, or professional care manager to ensure doctor's appointments are completed, healthy food is available, and good decisions are being made.	*It can become isolating. *Eating is a social experience. If eating alone, often little time is put into food preparation, and frozen and canned dinners become the staple. *Repairs on aging homes can draw down the available cash needed for living and future care expenses. *Unavailability of family members to help with transportation, yard work, and home maintenance can be a major variable in the long-term workability of this option. *Seniors become sedentary. *If the home and yard are not kept up, the senior may become a target for crime. *Costs for outside help can add up substantially. *Costs of property taxes can escalate, forcing seniors out of their homes.

Living options	Positives	Negatives
Move in with family	*Seniors often want the safety of living with family. *Lower levels of care can be provided, such as setting up medications, driving to doctor, food preparation, help with laundry, and housekeeping by family. * It is a way to reduce overall living costs.	*Role confusion: Family starts running the show. *Family life may be loud, ever-changing, not centered on the senior. *There may arise confusion about financial expectations. *Lonely: Everyone leaves for the day to work or school, leaving the parent home alone, maybe stranded, living in front of the TV.
Adult Day Care **Cost for week days only is $746**	Can provide daily care while family or spouse is at work or need respite from the care giving responsibilities.	*Care needs may exceed the ability of family to provide care 24/7 on an ongoing basis.

27

Living options	Positives	Negatives
Independent senior living apartments (55+) **Average rate $600-$1200/ month**	*These offer privacy, own kitchen, washer/dryer. *They may pay for some or all utilities. *Enjoy the company of other seniors. *Eliminate the weight of home ownership. *Pricing is at a lower rate than regular multifamily apartments.	*None have assisted living services for personal care needs. They don't address "aging in place" needs, so the senior may have to move as condition changes. *Often there is little management support on premises. No dining, housekeeping/linen, and transportation services may or may not be included. Activity programs are usually organized by the residents.

Living options	Positives	Negatives
Retirement community *Some retirement communities cater to the younger and/or healthier senior but also offer some personal care services, so residents can "age in place." *Other retirement communities do not offer personal care assistance, but seniors rely on home care companies or families. Typically, residents sign a month-to-month lease. Rates for the apartment cover all services except personal care services, i.e., medication management, assistance with bathing, dressing, grooming, escorts, transfers, etc. **Average rates $2500–$5000/month plus cost of care**	* Residents have their own private space, with their own kitchens and washer/dryer for personal laundry. *Lifestyle includes dining, housekeeping/linen services, transportation, and organized activities including exercise, learning, and entertainment. *Utilities, cable TV, Wi-Fi, and sometimes telephone services are included. *It includes closer observation of condition by staff in a non-intrusive way, which gives family and residents some peace of mind. (Typically, health indexes of seniors improve with more exercise, stimulation, and nutritional meals, and when they give up driving.)	*Can be expensive. But living at home is not necessarily free as many seniors will say (they tend to overlook the cost of yard and house maintenance, security services, property taxes, outside personal care costs, etc.). *Adjustment to community living may be a challenge for some.

29

Living options	Positives	Negatives
Assisted living community A pedestrian definition of assisted living is a little help every 3–4 hours. The costs of care are usually lower than professional home care services, which are one-on-one care, vs. a shared care program. **Average rates $3000–$5000/month plus cost of care per month*.** *A good resource is www. payingforseniorscare.com to help narrow average costs per area in the country. Typically, residents sign a month-to-month lease. Rates for the apartment cover all services except personal care services, i.e., medication management, assistance with bathing, dressing, grooming, escorts, transfers, etc.	*24-Hour assistance with ADLs is available. *Assisted living communities tend to address higher care needs (skin care, two person transfers, etc.). *They still have the privacy of their own apartment and are surrounded with their things. *These are regulated under state assisted living laws for safety reasons. *They may be able to offer diabetic care management (injections) with RN supervision.	*There are fewer activities to be involved in. *Costs can be much higher depending on care needed.
Adult family home (AFH) Resident has own room (not apartment) in a family home setting and typically shares meals with other residents. **Average rates $5000–$6500/month**	*Close supervision is provided. The senior can still enjoy a family-like environment vs. an institutional one. *Usually a high level of personal care is provided, i.e., feeding, mechanical lifts, etc. *Care is regulated by state for safety.	*Number of other residents may be only 4–6 people. Check state requirements. *Few activities are provided for residents, except the enjoyment of watching TV. *AFHs may have Medicaid contracts:

Living options	Positives	Negatives
Memory care community This is a variation on an assisted living community. Most states require that assisted living communities cannot use any form of restraint, i.e., locked doors, bed rails, certain levels of medication, etc.. So a senior has to have a diagnosis of dementia and prescription from their physician. Therefore, couples may be separated. **Average rates $5000-$7500/month**	*Secure (locked doors) environment to control for wandering out the doors. *Skilled staff are trained to deal with behavioral problems. *Most offer appropriate activities. *Residents with end stage dementia are offered high levels of personal assisted living care (incontinence care, full assist with bathing and dressing, feeding, etc.)	*These provide 24-hour supervision, so costs are high. *They may not be able to accommodate married couples living together.
Skilled nursing facility **Average rates $8000-12000/month**	Provides close supervision by medical professionals It provides advanced skilled care, such as, feeding tubes, infusions, injections, respiratory therapy, etc.	It offers institutional setting highly regulated resulting in rigid schedules and a less independent lifestyle. It can be extremely expensive.

*Lease rates are estimates and can vary with size of apartments, number of services and care included, as well as location (major or rural), market competitiveness, and economic conditions.

What's Important for Your Senior?

Here is a tool you can use first to evaluate the needs and preferences of your senior, lead the discussions with communities, discuss priorities with your senior, and then start to make a suitable match.

	Important	Not important	Not sure
Name of person:	**feature of lifestyle**	**feature**	
Size of community			
Number of events available every day including weekends			
Excursions outside the community (attending local theater, musicals, public gardens, museums, sporting events, casinos, etc.)			
Activities for people less physically able			
Activities for people less cognitively able			
Activities for people with high level of physical fitness			
Recognition of cultural or ethnic differences			
Activities to share with family			
Availability of religious events or celebrations			
Availability of lifelong learning events			
Availability of transportation			
Availability of all-day dining (open hours)			
Availability of open or assigned seating			
Number of options available on the menu			

Name of person:	Important feature of lifestyle	Not important feature	Not sure
Availability of special diet options (low salt, sugar free, gluten free, kosher)			
Availability of room service			
Option to accommodate people with low vision in the dining room			
Availability of valet service			
Availability of garden space to adopt			
Availability of overnight trips			
Resident feedback & ideas for activities program			
Availability of residents' evaluation of activity program, dining program			
Availability of aging in place (additional care)			
Permission for pets (is pet care available at an additional charge?)			
Permission for special laundry and cleaning products			

Touring

If staying in their home is no longer an option, here are some ideas to source living & care options for your loved one.

First you have to get educated. Fortunately, in today's market, it's easier to find what's out there. Looking on your favorite browser under "Retirement Communities", "Assisted Living", "Adult Family Homes", "Memory Care", or "Home Care Agencies" will generally provide a list of different organizations. Figuring out the best fit is the hard part.

Close family members or friends usually take on the role of searching out the best likely setting and care services for your loved one. However, logistics and urgency may dictate the need for professional assistance. There are private referral/placement agencies that will do the homework to provide a "short list" and guidance through the selection process. Their referral fees are usually paid by the operator of the community and not by the resident or resident's family. This can reduce a lot of frustration and time especially when parent's care needs are high. The downside is that the options they will suggest are generally only those communities that the referral agency has a contractual relationship with to pay the fee. You may miss out on great high occupancy communities that do not need to rely on these agencies for move-ins. But having a professional to expedite the process may be the right move for you. See Chapter 5 for help in sourcing these agencies.

Obviously finding a place that fits your senior now is the immediate goal, but you need to consider the best option that allows for some room to "age in place," thus avoiding another move right away. It is very hard to judge what is going to happen health-wise, but if a parent has a degenerate disease like Parkinson's, it is easier to map the likely challenges for the future, i.e., multiple number of staff available for transfers, mechanical lifts, etc. However, if a parent has a diagnosis of dementia but is still functioning at a high level (and is not wandering), it would be cruel to put them in a dementia care facility where people have end stage dementia.

Generally, I would recommend the family do the shopping before having "the talk" with your parent. After you have done your initial homework it's time to get them involved. Getting your senior active in the touring process is critical to getting their buy in, resulting in a competent decision and a higher quality of life after the move. Thoughtful tour planning is the key to success. For example, showing parents six retirement communities in a day will overwhelm them, delaying any decision-making for months. But showing them one or two will allow them to remember and discern whether the communities they just toured are a good fit.

Key Tour Questions:

- Rates of apartment-are there any features that add cost to base rent i.e. view, location in building

- Size of apartment-what amenities i.e. washer/dryer, baloney, fireplace, dish washer

   Determine what services are included in base rent: housekeeping, dining (how many meals per day), transportation (size of area), activities, utilities (which ones are included), Internet, emergency call system, telephone, cable TV, etc. What is refundable at move out? What if a resident runs out of money?

- Second occupant fee

   There is a monthly rental fee for a spouse, family member, or friend. This covers the costs for dining, transportation, activities, housekeeping etc. If the second person passes away or moves out, does the monthly rental rate decrease?

- Pet fee

   There may be a one-time fee or a monthly fee to address additional costs and wear and tear on the apartment. Typically, it is non-refundable, and if there is substantial damage to the apartment, there may be an additional charge at move out.

- Lease

   Is there a lease? If so, for how long? Is there a notice period for move out? Is the resident charged for a notice period if it is determined that the resident is no longer safe in the specific environment they are living in and is asked to move by the community? How much notice is required to vacate the apartment?

Most communities are month-to-month lease arrangements. Most require a thirty days' notice to vacate unless the community has determined that the person is no longer safe to live in the community. Once a given apartment has been chosen, a reservation fee may be charged. It may be a separate fee or go toward the move-in fee. There may be a move-in fee or community fee that is usually equal to one month's rent or less and is not refundable after move in. However, some communities offer a buy-in option, which also carries a monthly rental rate, often referred to as Continuing Care Retirement Communities (CCRCs) or Life Care Communities. The buy-in amount is typically substantial, in hundreds of thousands or six figure amounts, but a portion is usually refundable at move out.

- Rate of personal care

    Pricing assisted living care can be complicated. Assisted living is typically a function of time, i.e., how much time is needed to complete the task. Some communities charge for time of caregivers at one rate and time of licensed staff at another rate. Toileting, escorts, and dressing are often the most expensive in terms of time spent. Medication management can be time-consuming depending on the amount of medical monitoring that may be required (blood pressure, blood sugar, daily body weight, etc.).

    Care can be charged on a flat rate, level system, or on a point system basis.

    A flat rate charges everyone the same for the service. For example, medication management is charged at $400 per month. The problem is, Person A takes three medications two times a day, and Person B takes twenty-five medications five times a day. It's a good deal for Person B, as Person A is underwriting a portion of their care time.

A level system was created to be more flexible. Fc
some days if someone is experiencing a lot of pain,
or balance issue, a twenty-minute shower may take .
utes. If a person has a condition change or consister   ....s
longer time, then the senior may be moved up a level or two
to adjust for that. The problem is people are never really sure
what they are paying for.

Now that there are software programs, a point system is much
more granular, and it is a fair system as you pay for what you
use. It is a la-carte and well defined. So, in the case of the
example about medication assistance above, Person A will be
charged differently than Person B.

- How is a care plan developed?

    Is there an assessment charge? How often are they reassessed?
    Is the resident's physician required to determine if this person
    is safe behind a closed door in their apartment? How often
    is a person reassessed to note changes in condition, either
    improvement or decline? Clarify what would require a resi-
    dent to move out.

- What level of personal care is provided?

    1. With medication management the variables that go into
        providing that service include ordering medications, number
        of medications, and number of medication passes per day.
        Exceptions may exist if diabetic care management or injec-
        tions are given.

    2. Bathing, dressing, and grooming are standard services. Many
        seniors only need a little help with each of these. Others need
        full assistance. What about grooming (shaving assistance,
        salon services for cutting and styling hair, and manicures)?

3. Toileting, escorts, transfers, incontinence care are all examples of care.

*Toileting: Bladder incontinence care? Bowel incontinence care? Help to get to toilet and clean skin after? Who provides personal care products?

*Escorts: Assistance with walking or wheeled to the dining room and to activities?

*Transfers: One person or two person transfers? Mechanical lifts?

4. Dining: How many meals are included in the base rent if you are on assisted living services (many states require all three meals and snacks to be provided)? Are there menu options? Are there low-salt, sugar-free, gluten-free options? Can you accommodate low vision needs in the dining room? Do you have room service and what is the cost?

Here is a tool to use as you tour senior living communities:

Fill out form for each tour	Community: Location	Date
Key questions	Answers	Complete
Rates of apartment Size of apartments & amenities: washer/dryer, fireplace, balcony, dishwasher as well as view and location in the building. Services included in base rent: housekeeping, dining (how many meals per day), transportation (size of area), activities, etc. Utilities included: Internet, emergency call system, telephone, cable TV, etc. What is refundable at move out? What happens if a resident runs out of money?		
Second occupant fee Is there a monthly rental fee for a spouse, family member, or friend? What does it cover (costs for dining, transportation, activities, housekeeping, etc.)? If the second person passes away or moves out, does the monthly rental rate decrease?		

Fill out form for each tour	Community: Location	Date
Pet fee Monthly Rate? Is there a one-time fee or a monthly fee to address additional costs of wear and tear on the apartment? Is the fee non-refundable, and if there is substantial damage to the apartment, is there an additional charge at move out? Do you have pet care available? Grooming? Dog walking?		
Lease Is there a lease? If so, for how long? Is there a notice period for move out? Is the resident charged for a notice period if it is determined that the resident is no longer safe in this specific living environment and is asked to move by the community? How much notice is required to vacate the apartment?		
Rate for personal care What assistance with ADLs is available (medication management, dressing, grooming, toileting, transfers, escorts, etc.)? What care levels don't you do? When can a resident be asked to move?		

Fill out form for each tour	Community: Location	Date
How is the personal care plan developed? Who much does the assessment cost? Who does the assessment? Is one's doctor involved in the care planning process? How often is it reviewed? Will it change without sign off from family?		
Dining program How many meals are included in the base rent? Can you purchase additional meals? If so what is the cost of an extra meal or a month of daily three meals? Special diets? Guest meals?		
Transportation program Area of service? Costs for outside schedule and area?		

More questions

What is the staffing ratio (especially in care staff)?

What is the staff turnover?

What is the process for move-in?

Are there any promotions (free rent, moving expenses provided, waive pet fee)?

Is there a wait list (What is the likely wait time?)?

Is there a wait list fee (Does the fee expire? Is it refundable? If so, are there any provisions?)?

Ask for a copy of state survey, weekly menu/dining hours, and monthly activity calendar.

What charges are NOT included in the base rent or care charges?

Are there any other charges we have not discussed?

Do you have a money back guarantee?

The Fine Print

It can be helpful to pause and clarify some terms that can be misunderstood. It is not to suggest that a community is intentionally trying to mislead someone, but I have found areas of confusion over the years.

Twenty-four-hour Care

Here are some terms that are used but not always well defined. Assisted living services are services shared with others versus hiring a private caregiver. Assisted living is a little help every three to four hours, usually during the day, but caregivers are available twenty-four hours a day for caregiving (medication management, bathing, dressing, grooming, toileting, escorts, etc.). The cost of assisted living care is dramatically less than private duty care for the same services. Each resident has their own care plan that is directed by their physician and defined by the nurse.

Licensed Care

Licensed care is care provided directly by a licensed practical nurse or registered nurse. You can have the benefit of a more trained observer, who is more likely to recognize a change in condition earlier. These care professionals are highly trained and are therefore more expensive. In most states, only a registered nurse can produce a care plan by state law. However, many states have what is called nurse delegation. The registered nurse oversees the care plan and then trains caregivers to provide the care. The state nurse practice laws will determine who can do what. Regulations vary state to state so be sure to check with agencies in your jurisdiction.

Rehabilitation

Rehabilitation in a skilled nursing facility is done on an inpatient basis usually after a hospital stay. Once medically stabilized, a rehab facility can provide more close supervision and speech, physical, or occupational therapies. It is important to understand requirements in order for Medicare to pay for care. For example, a patient may have to be <u>admitted</u> (not just being observed) with a diagnosis and spend three midnights in the hospital. Clarify details with the social worker or discharge planner at the hospital. Daily rates in a rehab or skilled nursing facility can be over $700 per day.

Seniors often say that their greatest fear is ending up in a nursing home. A very small percentage of people today end up in a skilled nursing facility (formally known as a rest home) on a permanent basis. In fact, most skilled nursing facilities are retrofitting their operation to allocate their rooms to short-term rehabilitation versus permanent custodial care. It is amazing to see what rehab can accomplish with an eighty to ninety-year-old body! Many seniors want to dodge rehab after a hospital stay. They just want to go home. Depending on what the doctor says (of course), but typically this is a mistake. Home health therapies performed at the senior's home twice a week following hospitalization cannot compare to the daily intensive therapy received in a skilled nursing setting. If qualified, it is usually best to take advantage of this level of care.

The Safeguards

Because of the terrible abuse cases in nursing homes decades ago, this industry has become much more regulated by state agencies. For example, in the state of Washington, the Department of Social and Health Services is the regulatory agency with oversight to safeguard against senior neglect and abuse. The state does a surprise visit referred to as a survey every twelve to fifteen months by spending two to three days to inspect the safety, cleanliness, dignity, and wellbeing of residents. The current state surveys need to be posted for the public in the community and is available online on the website with the state agency. Home care, home health, referral agencies, assisted living, adult family homes, and skilled nursing homes are all regulated by state government.

How to Analyze If a Retirement Community is Alive and Well

Today's retirement communities are more like cruise ships than nursing homes. Yet, many seniors assume they are being put into a nursing home against their will, that it will smell bad, serve mashed peas, and all their daily choices will go away. Many nursing homes are not that way today either. The truth is, with the development of assisted living communities, less than 5 percent of seniors end up in a traditional nursing home on a permanent basis. *

*According to the US Census Bureau, about 4.2 **percent** of seniors are in **nursing homes** at any given time. Oct 21, 2011.

Measures of success would include the outcomes of the state surveys and the occupancy of the building. Most states require that communities post the outcomes of their last state survey. If not posted, ask for a copy or directions on how to get a copy.

What is considered a full community is around 98 percent occupied because there are move outs on an ongoing basis. The typical reasons people move out are (1) care needs exceed what can be provided, (2) passing away, or (3) to move closer to family. If the initial move-in process was done well, dissatisfaction and running out of money are far less frequent reasons for leaving!

Well-run communities have a defined inclusion process once a resident moves in. It is likely to include an opportunity to meet the department heads, other members of the *freshman class* (new residents), and a Buddy to escort them to the dining room or accompany them to an activity. Ask what would be done if your parent struggled to get connected in the community. Usually finding one friend is all that is needed to feel included.

If a given assisted living community or adult family home has a Medicaid contract, it is important that it is stipulated in the lease the conditions required to convert to the Medicaid program, i.e., length of stay, level of care, etc.

With the prevalence of social media, it's easy to get an inside look on resident satisfaction. Look for community reviews done by current and past residents, their families, and employees and vendors. It's getting harder and harder to hide. However, given there are no perfect places, understanding how resident concerns are addressed is critical to satisfaction.

Successful retirement communities typically deliver on what the doctor orders: stimulation, socialization, exercise, and nutritious good food. They offer a lifestyle to enhance their residents' safety and wellbeing.

Introducing families to the community lifestyle often produces the response "So how old does one have to be to move into one of these?" Having someone to clean your apartment, prepare your food, plan fun and activities for learning, sharing time with family, and developing new friends sounds pretty good to people of any age!

Each community has its own culture. Some are like neighborhoods, some like families, and others are more like clubs. Resident involvement is a measure of a healthy community, including a resident council, volunteer activities, and feedback through a Food, Dining, and Service Committee, an Activities Committee, or a Grounds and Garden Committee.

Three Levels of Resident Participation

1. Observation is standing on the sidelines. This passive level certainly can provide some stimulation and an opportunity to share with others.

2. Involvement is being on the court or playfield playing a certain role.

3. Engagement is the highest level of participation where people are involved and sharing their passion. At an engagement level, people experience a greater sense of aliveness, contribution, and joy. At the community where I worked, we strived to develop programs that engaged the residents with their passion, whether it was gardening, chorus, dance lessons, or painting pictures of shelter animals to promote pet adoptions and more.

Should I Stay or Should I go?

Keep in mind that at the end of the day, it's your parents' decision to stay at home or to go into senior living. Families can get in the way in a couple of ways. One is being overly excited, which can be experienced by your senior as being pushed! The other is pointing out all the things that you may prefer or not like. For example, a perfect apartment for the adult child may be an apartment with the view on the top floor down at the end of the hall. Where for the parent, it may be on the ground floor positioned across from the dining room. So, it is critical that everyone reflect back to what they say is important to them.

Chapter Four

The Talk, the Tour, the Timing

Most seniors go into retirement communities kicking and screaming, figuratively! We all love our homes, our yards, and most of all our memories. Leaving our homes and neighborhoods isn't easy for most. It can be uncomfortable, even fairly traumatic.

Let me tell you about what our family went through when it was time for this journey with my mother-in-law Susie.

Living in her condo, she was surrounded by seniors, she was on the board, and taking the two flights of stairs kept her in shape. But she had a couple of frightening experiences. One night a stranger followed her when she was out "pottying" her dog, and on another occasion, a stranger came to her door around 11:00 pm and tried to get in her door. So, she wanted to move to an apartment closer to her daughter and son's families.

We had tried to show her a retirement community at that juncture. Kaboom! She wouldn't get out of the car and she was convinced that we were dumping her off at an old-time nursing home. She was angry for weeks and it was an argument each time we brought it up. So we gave up and moved her into a multifamily apartment building. Most of those who lived there were young families or single, employed people who went off to work every day. Her life was sitting in her apartment all alone, disconnected!

Over time, we watched her go downhill. She became weepy, talked about dying, and though we as a family were with her three to five times a week, she spoke of being lonely. We finally said, "No more!" We picked the hill we were going to die on, all held hands, and said to her, "It's time." We reassured her that she can pick <u>where</u> she wanted to live if financially she could handle it. But she was moving! No negotiation on that. She finally entered the retirement community we wanted to show her before. She loved it and she lived there over five years. WHEW!

Six weeks after she moved into the retirement community, I bought her a new cobalt blue sweater with faux fur white collar. She put it on and modeled it in front of her mirror. She said, "This is going to drive the men crazy!" My husband and I smiled and said, "She's *baaaaack!*"

When moving into retirement communities, seniors aren't just changing houses but are moving into a new social situation that they haven't faced before. I liken it to going to college. Am I going to find friends? Are my clothes right? Will I embarrass myself?

We reframed the moving plan for my mother-in-law with all the children chanting, "Grandma is going to college!" She started giggling. We all, all twenty-six family members, stayed close and helped her move into her new apartment and life. The first evening she was frightened to go to the dining room by herself. Rightfully so…. A large dining room with one hundred people looking at you can be unnerving. But after a few days and help from the retirement community staff, she had regained her social confidence.

Within a couple of months, most residents are happy with the move and are getting after their children for not getting them moved sooner!

After they have made a couple of friends, things smooth out and they are on their way to another chapter of living. Keeping a positive end goal in mind, families can encourage confidence in your senior as they adapt to their new environment.-Most seniors successfully make the adjustment.

Some families are ready for battle and find that their parents have already made the decision. Some seniors are more educated by their friends' experience and privately do their own homework. It is a pleasurable experience to support one's parents' wishes to sell the family home and make a move into a retirement community where the family is assured that they are safe, stimulated, and enjoy the company of other seniors. But it is highly unlikely your senior will roll over that easy.

If you ask a senior if they want to move into a retirement community, they will most likely say, "Heck no!" What they hear is, "Do you want to move me into a community with a bunch of strangers, into a tiny apartment, and be told when to sleep and eat, what to wear, and be made to sing songs against my will?" OR, "My kids are trying to put me away in a stinky old nursing home like my grandmother lived in."

Get Ready, Get Set, Go . . .

Get Ready You have done your homework. Now it is important to match up real possibilities that are within your financial parameters.

Ask for referrals from friends and other trusted advisors. Get online and read reviews.

Get Set Go to your top two to three choices and preview these places and experience the staff and other residents.

Go!

The Talk

How do you frame the conversation? What are the steps to take when they refuse to go look? What are their fears? How do you get beyond the response, "I'm not ready"? Often a good question to ask in a kind way would be, "Mom what does 'ready' look like?"

Approach strategies to the talk:

- Addressing all the questions all at once is overwhelming. So start with "Where?" For the moment forget about "When". It may be a year from now.

- A very light-handed start is to simply leave some brochures around.

- If you can help them take one step, the next ones go easier and, in fact, many will get excited. A step may be dropping by a community after church.

- Getting your parents' physician to suggest a move to a retirement community can take things a long way.

- Engage a peer of your parents who has made it through the process and are glad they have done it. It can take a year or more for a senior to jump on the excitement program and go through the process. Unfortunately, unforeseen circumstances may require a more immediate move.

- Many times, selling a *Plan B* is better than pushing too hard to move right away.

I toured a son with his parents to introduce retirement living and show them an apartment within their budget. The son had joined the team in the corporate business office for the retirement community that I worked at. He realized that he needed to start a conversation with his parents about their future. His mother's caregiver (she had mobility issues) was his father, and his father had a heart condition. So, he finally persuaded his parents to come in. Through the tour they both were polite but assured me that they weren't ready and probably wouldn't be for a couple of years.

A couple of months later, his father developed pneumonia and passed away unexpectedly. His mother was devastated. After the funeral his mother said, "I am ready to move now." Having a plan helped her make a timely decision, create a safe nest where she could grieve the loss of her husband. And because she had to become more independent and more active, she became stronger psychologically and physically.

- Most people are overwhelmed with the question, "How am I going to be able to make all the decisions, dispose of all my stuff, and move everything?" Family members' reassurance is critical. Seniors' fear and expectation of themselves is they have to go through every box and piece of paper since 1973 before they can move. If the family can re-direct them to focus on <u>what they want to take with them going forward, it gets a whole lot easier very quickly.</u>

- Family support can really make the difference. I toured Mom, along with over fifteen family members that came to rally and support Mom. For some people that would not have worked, but for this family, everyone being there, asking the questions, tasting the food, and experiencing the community, put everyone on the same page and helped Mom face her future.

Chapter Five

Taking the Wheel

None of us know what lies ahead. We can try to predict based on the current look of things. For example, if someone has shown signs of Parkinson's, mobility issues or cognitive loss, they may be a predictor of what may be in one's future.

Our bodies and brains age differently. I visited Margaret, a ninety-six-year-old woman I've known for thirty years, in the hospital sometime back. She suffers from arthritis and overwhelming pain, but her clear-mindedness is amazing. I have also experienced Elsie, a 101-year-old woman, who lived a very physical life. Observing her walking, judging her gait, physical strength, and balance, one would swear she was in her seventies. Age is truly relevant!

Decisions That Have to be Made

Getting answers to some important questions can reassure seniors that their house is in order. So, long before moving decisions are made, it's important to ask some important questions. These questions need to be discussed with other trusted advisors including one's banker, financial planner, accountant, and lawyer.

- Who is going to make decisions about their care and use of their finances if they are not able? (Decisions that reflect their preferences and wishes)

- What if their appointed representatives are not reachable?

- Who will act on their behalf if they find someone has proven to be acting irresponsibly?

- What are their rights under the law?

The Paperwork

- Power of attorney healthcare

- Power of attorney for finance

- Guardianship, produced through the courts

- Advanced directives

- POLST forms

- Five wishes

When preparing a will, often there are associated documents that reflect the answer to who is going to act on behalf of the senior. Wills become out of date, and laws change from one state to another. So, it is important to ensure directives are up to date. Beyond the distribution of the estate's assets, a personal representative (formally called an executor) is named to ensure the distribution reflects the <u>deceased</u> person's wishes after death. But before death, who will ensure a living senior's wishes are fulfilled?

Many times, seniors who are not able will appoint one or two different members of their family to guide decision-making. These are revocable and are very limited. If a senior is not capable of making decisions established by a physician and/or there has been evidence of nefarious actions by a power of attorney or there are no family members capable or available to safeguard the older adult, a guardian is appointed by the court.

Documents that outline the actions that someone wants or doesn't want during a medical emergency are referred to as advance directives. The problem is that most wills are stored in a safety deposit box in their bank or a safe in their home. This is not very handy during an emergency.

The US medical community has proposed using a universal form that is signed by a physician to govern the decision of medical intervention. In the state of Washington, medical professionals will only recognize a POLST form (Physician Order for Life-Sustaining Treatment), or else they will administer resuscitation. It is suggested that the POLST form be posted on the front door, fridge, or bathroom door so that emergency personnel can quickly access the information they need to respond to your advance directives. *https://polst.org/programs-in-your-state/

A wonderful document produced by Aging with Dignity called Five Wishes is a great tool to facilitate this discussion. *www.agingwithdignity. org.

Who Else Can Help?
There are other situations where families need an extra set of hands to work through the process of getting their parent/s into a safe place quickly.

- What if Mom and Dad live three thousand miles away? How to take care of them from here? In today's world, it is not uncommon that adult children face this reality across the country.

- Many have their own health issues, family, and/or jobs that require all their attention.

- Or what if their parent ends up in the hospital and doctors have made the decision to not discharge the parent to their home after their stay and now you have twenty-four to forty-eight hours to figure it all out?

Geriatric Care Managers: Care managers can help facilitate decision-making and taking actions to get your senior the help they need. These professionals are licensed and/or certified to perform these services. There are a growing number of professionals that can help manage or implement assessments, moves, admissions, flights, etc. They are a fee-based service. https://www.aginglifecare.org/

Move Managers: What if your parent lives across the country? There are transition companies that will manage the packing, moving, unpacking, and selling personal items and/or property that is no longer needed. They are also a fee-based service. https://www.nasmm.org/

Referral Companies: There are professionals that can provide you a list of vetted adult family homes, retirement communities, assisted living communities, memory care communities, and skilled nursing facilities. Some offer more hands-on services where they escort you to tour properties, and others are more of a clearing house. Their services are free to the senior and their family, with fees paid by the provider.

In Washington State: http://www.asrpwa.org/2018-member-list/

National Placement & Referral Alliance (formed in 2017) http://www.npralliance.org

Realtors with Senior Certifications: A specialized service now being provided by some real estate brokerages serves to address the special issues that seniors face when making this life transition. https://sres.realtor/work-sres-designee/find-member

Chapter Six

How Grandma Got Swindled!
How to Protect Your Parent

Seniors today are educated enough to know better than to give that smooth talker on the other end of the phone their social security number, bank account number, or credit card number. However, there continues to be a stream of situations, phone calls, mail requests from phony sweepstakes, political contributions to save the free world, and charity contribution requests. A recent Investor Protection Trust survey found that one in every five seniors, aged sixty-five or older, has been financially duped! *www.moneymanagement.org/blog/...financial-elder-abuse.aspx

Bob, with his son, had come to look into retirement living. He didn't move in right away but would drop by from time to time. His son honored his father's process and didn't push him. But he became concerned when his father became secretive about his money. He had said that he had made some investments and was waiting to get his pay out.

Bob had asked if it was okay to have his girlfriend move in with him as he wasn't ready to get married. The son was curious about who his girlfriend was. Dad said she lived in Europe but wanted to come and be with him. Finally, the son figured out that his father had sent over $250,000 to this woman for investment. Bob would not accept that he had been robbed. The son decided that it would be safer to get his father out of his house, change his phone number, and put some protections in place to prevent him from sending more money to this woman. Bob moved into our community, and within the first week he re-contacted his *girlfriend* (whom he had not met in person) and sent another $7000! The son finally set up three bank accounts each with limited funds. Bob could feel like he had control over the bills and worked with the banker to be notified about any large money transfer requests. Bob's story may be an extreme example but this type of fraud does occur. However, the more likely-to-happen scenario is hiding in plain sight—families abuse their role as a power of attorney (people given, in good faith, privileges by the senior to act on their behalf).

Exploitation can be very subtle. Two family members of a family of five adult children took me aside with concerns that their other three unemployed siblings were sneaking into their dad's retirement community apartment through the back door and spending nights with dear old Dad. They assumed that they could stay rent free with Dad. Their father would bring in food from the dining room to feed them and certainly didn't want to kick them out. But the other siblings were concerned as this would be considered elder abuse, with Dad and his resources caring for his adult children. Typically, communities have a time frame of two to three weeks for visitors to stay over. Otherwise they are considered taking up residency and need to sign a lease.

I have also witnessed a resident's friend, after having sold her home, come to have lunch with the resident. Jean had invited her friend to come spend a couple of nights in her apartment because it was a couple hour drive back to where her friend had lived. Pretty soon it became evident to Jean that her friend was planning a much longer stay, rent-free, of course!

Jean panicked and came to me for help. We respectfully treated her friend like a guest but clarified the ground rules.

Families, friends, and even professionals can be a great service to seniors by taking over the bills and finances. But it can also let the fox into the hen house. Older adults need to have copies of all bank statements, credit cards, and investment accounts and insist that they participate in all discussions with bankers, attorneys, and realtors.

Grooming

Fraud victimization of older adults includes using fear and abusing their sense of dependency by telling them how lucky they are to have this help. For example, a gentleman, Tim, didn't have any family and was trying to decide if he should to move into the retirement community. He was lonely, and his only friends were from his church. Tim's minister had accompanied him to act on his "flock's" behalf. He moved in, adjusted well, and seemed to enjoy his new lifestyle. About six months later, Tim decided to move out. It turned out that Tim had actually moved into his minister's new home, in which Tim had invested some of his money. After moving out, Tim would come by and say hello. Tim was home alone most days and was feeling pretty isolated. Unfortunately, his resources were tied up in this home purchase, which prevented him from moving back to the community where there were activities and friends his own age. The ElderCare Rights Alliance outlines common tactics abusers use to gain control. www. eldercarerights.org.

If you suspect any neglect or abuse, there are several resources that can help with investigation and legal protection.

- Adult family homes, assisted living communities, and skilled nursing facilities have the Long-Term Care Ombudsman Program, which is federally funded. Ombudsmen are trained and act as a non-paid, third party to advocate for the residents' needs.

- In Washington state, Adult Protective Services is a state agency that will investigate and take legal action if there is a basis for fraud and abuse.

National Bank of Mom and Dad

Most parents help their family financially at one time or another. Personal loans with no signed IOU paperwork outlining the terms and conditions of the loan can become a source of conflict if not litigation. Verbal agreements can get lost in the confusion of everyday life. Memory of discussions may not reflect the original intentions. Writing something down allows more discussion for a clear expectation. If you are responsible for managing the finances for your parents be sure to keep documentation for all transactions as you can be held legally responsible.

Financial planners suggest that seniors should watch out for their own needs rather than pay for their grandchildren's college or pay down payment on their children's new house. Those funds should be used to provide the needed funds for the senior's care to relieve families of that burden. There are funds to go to college: scholarships, grants, and student loans. But there are no loans for seniors to pay for their care.

A Prominent Area for Theft

Street value medications (narcotics) are frequently stolen from seniors. Assisted living communities have procedures to control for theft of medication. When the assisted living department is taking the responsibility for distributing the medications, narcotics are counted at the beginning of the shift and the end of the shift. If someone is handling their own medications, communities often provide or are required to provide locked cabinets to secure their medications.

Chapter Seven

Joining Their Journey

This life change can be an energizing and positive experience for all. Mom may want some new clothes or a new hairstyle to boost her confidence. Purchasing new furniture can also encourage socializing and inviting new friends into their apartment. Hosting an open house for old neighbors and friends or for people living on their wing or floor can help them embrace the change with excitement.

If a senior is struggling with some early dementia, changing all their furniture and furnishings may not be a good idea. Familiarity is comforting. In fact, laying out the furniture in the living room and bedroom similar to their home is helpful. Having Mom unpack her own kitchen the way it makes sense to her will help her be able to find things in the future.

Having a family member spend the first couple of nights with them in their apartment and escorting them to meals can reduce some of the initial social anxiety.

Many communities have resident ambassadors that reach out to new people, accompany them to meals and community events, introduce them to others, and explain the rules of the road. Inquire about new resident orientations where they can meet other *members of the freshmen class*, the department heads, and learn how they can get their continuing questions answered.

A New Chapter

Taking a couple class, going to bingo, ~~or~~ and doing a day trip offered by the community a couple of weeks after moving in, may be a stretch. Family members may need to accompany your senior to activities the first time. ~~But~~ Keep it simple. Doing just one activity will help them meet people.

Understanding that your parent(s) may not feel on the top of their power curve is crucial. Listening, reassurance, and encouragement tend to soften the fear, and then over time this new place becomes home. This could take up to six months.

Having the weight of housework and cooking off their backs, seniors are freed up to spend time doing the things they love. Many people find they sleep better, eat better, and even exercise. Sharing common history, music, and humor with others aids in creating a sense of belonging. Seeing other seniors conquer iPhones, doing yoga, and writing down their life story gives them things to share with their family members in a new way.

Although infrequent, some even make new love connections. Some come out of the closet. And some finally start actively pursuing their bucket list. It's never too late!

One of the most memorable events that was inspired by our Activity Director, Dora, was Wedding Day. Historically residents brought down their wedding pictures that were displayed during the month of June for others to enjoy. This particular year she overheard some residents discussing the fact that they didn't have a white wedding. After the war, resources were scarce. So most got married in a lovely suit, but it was not the same.

So, Dora went to work on it. She planned a Wedding Day for seven residents. She called out to staff to loan out their own wedding dresses and went to a bridal shop that loaned some white bridal gowns for the day. Families and staff were asked to escort the brides down the aisle to the sounds of the Wedding March.

Everyone got their hair and makeup done, bridal bouquets were made, and the photographers were ready. The procession was followed with a reception with a tiered wedding cake, wine, and love songs from the 40s and 50s.

The joy, the tears, the outer beauty, and the inner peace brought out by this event were unmatched to any other event. *"At Last . . ."*

A Legacy

One of highest levels of human development is the knowledge than one has left a mark on the planet, knowing they have made an impact on others' lives. What is a legacy? "Often when you think about legacy, it's something that is left behind after a person has passed. Legacy is more about sharing what you have learned, not just what you have earned, and bequeathing values over valuables, as material wealth is only a small fraction of your legacy." *Meridian Life Designs, Inc., Life Coaching and Legacy Coaching Services, West Vancouver, BC Canada.

Capturing your parents' thoughts and learnings for future generations can serve their sense of having lived a worthy life.

I have always believed in intergenerational interaction for the learning that takes place. The principal of a nearby high school and I sponsored a co-learning experience for Juniors and Seniors in social study classes and some of our interested residents. The focus was the Great Depression. Students were required to read one hundred pages, look at one hundred images, and for one hundred minutes talk to an older adult that had lived through it We started with sixty students and fifteen seniors.

Word got out, and an additional forty students joined in to hear the well-crafted questions from the social studies teacher and answers from our panel of *experts*: "How did you know there was a depression going on?" "Did you live in the city, a village, or a farm?" "How was your family impacted?" "What did you do to survive?"

Students were riveted and loved hearing the answers. They learned about the Dust Bowl, the Roosevelts, soup lines, and how people put old newspapers in their shoes to prevent their feet from getting wet because of the holes in their shoes.

In the follow-up session, students presented their learnings. In multimedia presentations to the seniors, they included music and images of The Depression years.

In a debrief with our participating residents, they reported being in awe of the quality of these students represented. In fact, these were public school students, not necessarily honor students or handpicked to be there. The magic happened because people were authentic, respectful, and excited about the human experience.

I share these examples to demonstrate the kind of legacy experiences your loved one may choose to have as a resident in a quality senior living community. There can be much to look forward to for the senior and your entire family. Families can create legacy discussions and experiences as well.

Chapter Eight

Saying Goodbye

The *2009 Overview of Assisted Living* reported the average stay in assisted living communities is twenty-eight months! That's a lot to come to terms with as a family. Of course, it is a case-by-case situation. As sobering as it is, it's a time when everyone involved should strive to make it the best twenty eight months possible. * www.ahcancal.org

The joy of parents that have lived across the country for decades and are now able to see their children four to five days a week knows no bounds. This is the time to sit with them, with your arm around them, and giggle about the crazy times and listen to the stories that you have heard hundreds of times. But maybe it's more about the chance you get to see through and listen beyond the words and peek into their hearts and souls. You will be so glad that you did.

Knowing the end is near and discussing the end together can bring great comfort. In the Five Wishes exercise mentioned earlier, the best gift one can give to their family and friends is telling them what you want them to know. My minister said that people are often most alive as they get closer to death. Finding grace to accept each other with the flaws we all have and celebrating what you shared can bring peace.

We don't always get to know ahead of time as in my mother's case. She lived in southern Saskatchewan near my brothers. She had emphysema, but overall she was doing pretty well until she got pneumonia. One Easter, I got a call from my brother saying our mother didn't have much time. So, we got on the next available plane, caught another connecting flight, rented a car, and missed the border crossing from Montana into Canada by five minutes. We finally got to her assisted living community early the next day. Luckily, she was aware enough to know I was there. My mother was a Godly woman and believed in receiving last rights. So, I tried to track down the minister that had been calling on her over the last couple of years. I finally reached him over phone and told him about my mother's state and asked if he could come and visit with her. He said he wasn't available and said he would come the next day.

Being a former nurse, I could see her body was slowly shutting down and feared she would not be with us the next day. I realized that I had to give her last rights. Clumsily, I took her hand and prayed with her about forgiveness and being forgiving. We blessed and thanked her for her love, sacrifice, and commitment to our family.

I, then, gave her permission to go to the light, her Jesus Christ, knowing we were fine. It was her time. She died a couple of minutes later. I came into the world in her arms and she went out in mine. What a wonderful gift that I am so thankful for!

It is my hope that you too can have a special final Goodbye with your loved one.

Chapter Nine

Your Turn

There is no better time than now for adult children to get their own house in order.

One of the big lessons adult children learn is having things in order reduces a lot of anxiety and unnecessary worry. One of the best gifts you can give your family is having your ducks in a row. The last few pages of this book will help you with that effort.

Warmest regards!

Get Your Ducks in a Row

Date_____

Name _____

Nick Name _____

MaidenName _____

Address _____

Phone Number _____

Cell _____

Work _____

Email _____

Date of Birth _____

Birthplace _____

Social Security Number _____

Medicare Number _____

Power of Attorney for Health Care _____

Contact Information _____

Power of Attorney for Finances Contact Information ____

Emergency Contacts _____

Contact 1 _____

Relationship _____

Contact 2 _____

Contact Information _____

Relationship _____

Health Insurance _____

      Number _____

Company _____

        Phone _____

Long-term-care Insurance _____

      Number _____

Company _____

      Phone _____

Primary Care Physician

Name _____

Clinic _____

Address _____

Phone _____

Specialists

Name _____

Specialty _____

Clinic _____

Address _____

Phone _____

Name _____

Specialty _____

Clinic _____

Address _____

Phone _____

Name _____

Specialty _____

Clinic _____

Address _____

Phone _____

Hospital Preference _____

Address _____

Retirement Community Preference _____

Address _____

Dentist

Name _____

Clinic _____

Address _____

Phone _____

Eye Doctor

Name _____

Specialty _____

Clinic _____

Address _____

Phone _____

Quick Facts _____

Veteran Yes _____ No _____

If yes, military service number _____

Branch _____ Years of service_____ Discharge papers_____

Storage location _____

Circle as many as are relevant:

Blind   Hard of hearing   Use a cane or walker   Use a wheelchair

Glasses   Contact lenses   Dental appliance   Pacemaker

Defibrillator   Prosthesis   Hearing aid

Will   Living will   Advance directive   POLST form

Organ donor Yes _____ No _____

Blood type   A   B   AB   O   Positive Negative

Medical History:

Diagnosis:

_____

_____

_____

List of Surgeries:

Surgery _____Where _____

Date_____

Surgery _____Where _____

Date_____

Surgery _____Where _____

Date_____

Hospice Care Provider

Location _____

Phone_____

List of Medications

Pharmacy _____

Address _____

Phone Number _____

Medication _____

Ailment _____

Last Date Updated _____

Medication _____

Ailment _____

Last Date Updated _____

Medication _____

Ailment _____

Last Date Updated _____

Medication _____

Ailment _____

Last Date Updated _____

Medication _____

Ailment _____

Last Date Updated _____

Medication _____

Ailment _____

Bank _____

Account _____

Address _____

Phone _____

Bank _____

Account _____

Address _____

Phone _____

Bank _____

Account _____

Address _____

Phone _____

FinancialPlanner/Broker _____

Account _____

Address _____

Phone _____

Insurance Broker _____

Address _____

Phone _____

Accountant _____

Address _____

Phone _____

Member of a Church Yes _____ No _____

Denomination _____

Address _____

Clergy's Name _____

Phone _____

Funeral Home _____

FuneralHomeDirector _____

Address _____

Phone _____

Arrangements Made

Burial plot   Yes _____   No _____

If yes, location _____

Plot purchased Yes_____No_____

Funeral Service Preferences

Location _____

Officiate _____

Readings _____

Music _____

Participants_____